AF420134

The Real Key to Gut Health: The Gut, Heart and Brain Connection

Prologue:

Have you ever experienced gut discomfort, only to find that your mood and energy levels also suffer? Or have you struggled with a heart condition, only to realize that it may be linked to your gut health? The connection between our gut, heart, and brain is more complex and interrelated than we once thought.

The gut, often referred to as our "second brain," plays a crucial role in our overall health and well-being. It's not just about digestion, but also about how our gut health affects our immune system, mood, and even our heart health.

In this book, we'll explore the gut-heart-brain connection and how taking care of our gut can improve our heart and brain health. We'll delve into the latest research on gut health, the role of probiotics and prebiotics, and the benefits of an elimination diet. We'll also discuss the potential dangers of a high-fiber diet and the benefits of a carnivore diet.

By the end of this book, you'll have a deeper understanding of the gut-heart-brain connection and the impact that gut health has on our overall health. Whether you're a healthcare professional or simply someone looking to improve your health, this book will provide you with the knowledge and tools to take control of your gut health and lead a happier, healthier life.

Chapter 1: Discovering the Cause of Gut Health Issues

In recent years, the connection between gut health and overall health has become increasingly recognized. The gut has been dubbed the "second brain" due to its complex network of nerves and its impact on both physical and mental health. In this chapter, we will explore the connection between gut health, the heart, and the brain, and why it's crucial to prioritize gut health for overall wellbeing.

The Importance of Gut Health:

The gut is home to trillions of bacteria, fungi, and viruses, collectively known as the gut microbiome. These microorganisms play a crucial role in maintaining a healthy gut and influencing various functions in the body, including the immune system, digestion, and mental health. An imbalance in the gut microbiome, known as dysbiosis, has been linked to various health problems, such as inflammation, digestive issues, and mood disorders.

The Gut-Heart Connection:

Studies have shown that there is a direct link between gut health and heart health. The gut microbiome can influence heart health by regulating blood pressure, cholesterol levels, and inflammation in the body. A healthy gut can also help reduce the risk of heart disease and stroke.

The Gut-Brain Connection:

The gut and brain are connected through the gut-brain axis, a network of nerves and signaling pathways. The gut microbiome can influence brain function by producing neurotransmitters, such as serotonin and dopamine, which play a role in mood and behavior. A healthy gut can help improve mental health and reduce the risk of depression and anxiety.

In conclusion, the connection between gut health, the heart, and the brain is complex and far-reaching. Maintaining a healthy gut is crucial for overall health and wellbeing. In subsequent chapters, we will explore the various ways to support gut health, including diet, lifestyle, and probiotics. By prioritizing gut health, we can improve our physical and mental health, and reduce the risk of various health problems.

Chapter 2: The Role of Diet in Gut Health

Introduction:

One of the most important factors in maintaining a healthy gut is diet. The foods we eat can directly impact the composition of the gut microbiome, influencing its diversity and balance. In this chapter, we will explore the role of diet in gut health, and how certain foods and nutrients can support a healthy gut and reduce the risk of dysbiosis.

The Impact of Processed Foods:

Processed foods, such as junk food and sugary snacks, have been linked to an increased risk of gut dysbiosis and inflammation. These foods can disrupt the balance of the gut microbiome, leading to an overgrowth of harmful bacteria and a decrease in beneficial bacteria.

The Benefits of Fiber:

Fiber is essential for gut health, as it provides food for the gut microbiome and helps regulate digestion. Foods high in fiber, such as fruits, vegetables, and whole grains, have been shown to support a healthy gut and reduce the risk of dysbiosis.

Fermented Foods:

Fermented foods, such as yogurt, kefir, and sauerkraut, are rich in probiotics, which are beneficial bacteria that support gut health. Consuming fermented foods can help to increase the diversity of the gut microbiome, improving its balance and reducing the risk of dysbiosis.

Prebiotics:

Prebiotics are non-digestible fibers that serve as food for the gut microbiome. Foods high in prebiotics, such as garlic, onions, and bananas, have been shown to support a healthy gut and improve gut function.

Conclusion:

In conclusion, diet plays a crucial role in gut health. By focusing on a diet that is rich in fiber, fermented foods, and prebiotics, and avoiding processed foods, we can support a healthy gut and reduce the risk of dysbiosis. In subsequent chapters, we will explore additional ways to support gut health, including lifestyle and probiotics. By prioritizing gut health, we can improve our physical and mental wellbeing.

Chapter 3: Lifestyle Factors in Gut Health

Introduction:

In addition to diet, lifestyle factors such as stress, sleep, and physical activity also play a crucial role in gut health. In this chapter, we will explore the impact of lifestyle factors on the gut microbiome and how they can be used to support a healthy gut and reduce the risk of dysbiosis.

The Impact of Stress:

Stress has been shown to have a negative impact on the gut microbiome, leading to an imbalance in its composition. Chronic stress can also lead to an overgrowth of harmful bacteria, and can contribute to the development of digestive problems and mental health disorders.

The Importance of Sleep:

Sleep is essential for overall health, and it also plays an important role in gut health. Lack of sleep has been linked to gut dysbiosis, inflammation, and an increased risk of digestive problems. Aiming for 7-9 hours of quality sleep per night can help to support a healthy gut and improve overall wellbeing.

Physical Activity:

Physical activity has been shown to have a positive impact on the gut microbiome, increasing its diversity and promoting the growth of beneficial bacteria. Regular exercise can also help to reduce stress and improve sleep, which are both crucial factors in maintaining a healthy gut.

The Benefits of Relaxation Techniques:

Relaxation techniques, such as mindfulness and yoga, have been shown to have a positive impact on the gut microbiome. These techniques can help to reduce stress and improve sleep, supporting a healthy gut and reducing the risk of dysbiosis.

Conclusion:

In conclusion, lifestyle factors play a crucial role in gut health. By focusing on stress reduction, adequate sleep, physical activity, and relaxation techniques, we can support a healthy gut and reduce the risk of dysbiosis. By prioritizing gut health, we can improve our physical and mental wellbeing and reduce the risk of various health problems. In subsequent chapters, we will explore additional ways to support gut health, including probiotics. By incorporating diet, lifestyle, and probiotics into our daily routine, we can optimize our gut health and achieve overall wellbeing.

Chapter 4: The Gut-Heart-Brain Connection

Introduction:

The gut, heart, and brain are interconnected through complex signaling pathways, and the health of one can directly impact the health of the others. In this chapter, we will explore the gut-heart-brain connection, and how maintaining a healthy gut can improve heart health and brain function.

The Gut and Heart Health:

Studies have shown that the gut microbiome has a significant impact on heart health. A healthy gut microbiome is associated with a lower risk of cardiovascular disease, while an imbalance in the gut microbiome has been linked to an increased risk of heart disease. The gut microbiome can affect heart health by influencing inflammation, cholesterol levels, and blood pressure.

The Gut and Brain Function:

The gut microbiome has also been shown to play a role in brain function. The gut microbiome can impact brain health by producing neurotransmitters, influencing inflammation, and impacting the blood-brain barrier. A healthy gut microbiome is associated with improved mood and cognitive function, while an imbalance in the gut microbiome has been linked to an increased risk of depression, anxiety, and neurodegenerative diseases.

Conclusion:

In conclusion, the gut-heart-brain connection highlights the importance of maintaining a healthy gut. By prioritizing gut health through a balanced diet, lifestyle factors, and probiotics, we can improve heart health, brain function, and overall wellbeing. In subsequent chapters, we will explore additional ways to support gut health, including probiotics and supplements. By making gut health a priority, we can impact multiple aspects of our health and improve our overall wellbeing.

Chapter 5: Supporting Gut Health with Probiotics and Supplements

Introduction:

In addition to diet and lifestyle, probiotics and supplements can also play a role in supporting gut health and reducing the risk of dysbiosis. In this chapter, we will explore the benefits of probiotics and supplements, and how they can be used to support a healthy gut.

The Benefits of Probiotics:

Probiotics are beneficial bacteria that can help to support a healthy gut by promoting the growth of beneficial bacteria and reducing the growth of harmful bacteria. Probiotics have been shown to have a number of health benefits, including improving digestive function, reducing inflammation, and improving mood and cognitive function. Probiotics can be found in fermented foods such as yogurt, kefir, and kimchi, or can be taken in supplement form.

The Benefits of Prebiotics:

Prebiotics are a type of fiber that feed the beneficial bacteria in the gut. By promoting the growth of beneficial bacteria, prebiotics can help to support a healthy gut and reduce the risk of dysbiosis. Prebiotics can be found in foods such as bananas, onions, garlic, and asparagus, or can be taken in supplement form.

Supplements for Gut Health:

In addition to probiotics and prebiotics, there are other supplements that can help to support gut health. Supplements such as glutamine, vitamin D, and omega-3 fatty acids have been shown to have a positive impact on gut health. However, it is important to talk to a healthcare professional before starting any new supplement regimen.

Conclusion:

In conclusion, probiotics and supplements can play a role in supporting gut health and reducing the risk of dysbiosis. By incorporating a balanced diet, lifestyle factors, probiotics, and supplements into our daily routine, we can optimize our gut health and achieve overall wellbeing. It is important to talk to a healthcare professional before starting any new supplement regimen to ensure that they are safe and appropriate for your individual needs. By prioritizing gut health, we can improve our physical and mental wellbeing and reduce the risk of various health problems.

Chapter 6: The Vagus Nerve and the Gut-Heart-Brain Connection

Introduction:

The vagus nerve is a critical component of the gut-heart-brain connection, and plays a crucial role in regulating the health of these three organs. In this chapter, we will explore the role of the vagus nerve in the gut-heart-brain connection and how it can be used to support overall health.

The Role of the Vagus Nerve:

The vagus nerve is the longest of the cranial nerves, and runs from the brainstem to the abdomen. The vagus nerve is responsible for controlling various bodily functions, including digestion, heart rate, and immune function. It also plays a role in regulating mood and cognitive function.

The Vagus Nerve and the Gut:

The vagus nerve is critical for the regulation of digestive function, and is responsible for controlling the release of digestive juices and the contraction of the muscles in the gut. A healthy vagus nerve can help to ensure optimal digestive function, while a compromised vagus nerve can lead to digestive problems such as constipation, bloating, and heartburn.

The Vagus Nerve and the Heart:

The vagus nerve also plays a role in regulating heart rate and blood pressure. By slowing down the heart rate, the vagus nerve can help to reduce stress and improve heart health. This is why techniques such as deep breathing and meditation, which stimulate the vagus nerve, can be beneficial for heart health.

The Vagus Nerve and the Brain:

The vagus nerve also plays a role in regulating mood and cognitive function. By reducing inflammation and promoting the release of neurotransmitters, the vagus nerve can help to improve mood and cognitive function. Techniques such as deep breathing, meditation, and yoga can be used to stimulate the vagus nerve and improve brain function.

Conclusion:

In conclusion, the vagus nerve plays a critical role in the gut-heart-brain connection, and is a key component of overall health. By promoting a healthy vagus nerve through techniques such as deep breathing, meditation, and yoga, we can improve digestive function, heart health, and brain function. In addition, incorporating probiotics and supplements into our daily routine can help to further support the health of the vagus nerve and the gut-heart-brain connection. By prioritizing the health of the vagus nerve, we can improve our overall wellbeing and reduce the risk of various health problems.

Chapter 7: Step 1, Gut Health

Introduction:

In recent years, the connection between gut health and overall health has become increasingly recognized, and it is now widely accepted that the health of the gut plays a crucial role in the health of the heart and brain. In this chapter, we will explore why gut health is the most important part of the gut-heart-brain connection.

The Gut as the Foundation of Health:

The gut is often referred to as the "second brain" due to the complex network of nerves that run from the gut to the brain. The gut is also home to trillions of bacteria, which play a critical role in maintaining overall health. A healthy gut is essential for a healthy immune system, as well as for the proper digestion and absorption of nutrients.

The Connection between Gut Health and Heart Health:

Studies have shown that a healthy gut can help to reduce the risk of heart disease. This is because the gut is responsible for producing hormones that regulate blood pressure and cholesterol levels, and for removing harmful substances from the body. A healthy gut can also help to reduce inflammation, which is a major risk factor for heart disease.

The Connection between Gut Health and Brain Health:

The gut and brain are connected through the gut-brain axis, which is a complex network of nerves and hormones that regulate the communication between the gut and brain. A healthy gut can help to improve mood and cognitive function, as well as reduce the risk of neurological conditions such as depression, anxiety, and Alzheimer's disease.

The Importance of a Balanced Microbiome:

The gut microbiome is made up of trillions of bacteria, and a healthy gut microbiome is essential for overall health. A balanced microbiome can help to improve digestion, boost the immune system, and reduce the risk of chronic diseases. However, an imbalanced microbiome can lead to digestive problems, immune dysfunction, and an increased risk of chronic diseases.

Conclusion:

In conclusion, gut health is the most important part of the gut-heart-brain connection, as it lays the foundation for overall health. A healthy gut is essential for reducing the risk of heart disease, improving brain function, and maintaining a balanced microbiome. By prioritizing gut health through a healthy diet, regular exercise, and stress management, we can improve our overall health and reduce the risk of various health problems. Additionally, incorporating probiotics and supplements into our daily routine can help to further support the health of the gut and the gut-heart-brain connection. By focusing on gut health, we can improve our overall wellbeing and achieve optimal health.

Chapter 8: Why You Should Care About the Gut-Heart-Brain Connection

Introduction:

In this chapter, we will explore the numerous benefits of a healthy gut-heart-brain connection. A healthy gut has a significant impact on overall health, and by prioritizing gut health, we can improve the health of our heart and brain, as well as our overall wellbeing.

Improved Heart Health:

A healthy gut can help to reduce the risk of heart disease by regulating blood pressure and cholesterol levels, reducing inflammation, and removing harmful substances from the body. A healthy gut also supports a strong immune system, which can help to protect against heart disease.

Improved Brain Health:

A healthy gut can also improve brain health by reducing the risk of neurological conditions such as depression, anxiety, and Alzheimer's disease. The gut-brain axis, the complex network of nerves and hormones that regulate the communication between the gut and brain, is essential for maintaining brain health. A healthy gut can help to improve mood, cognitive function, and memory.

Reduced Inflammation:

Inflammation is a major risk factor for chronic diseases, including heart disease, neurological conditions, and autoimmune diseases. A healthy gut can help to reduce inflammation by producing hormones that regulate inflammation and by maintaining a balanced microbiome.

Improved Digestion and Absorption of Nutrients:

A healthy gut can help to improve digestion and the absorption of nutrients, which is essential for overall health. A balanced microbiome can help to break down food, absorb nutrients, and eliminate waste, while an imbalanced microbiome can lead to digestive problems and nutrient deficiencies.

Improved Immune System:

The gut is home to trillions of bacteria, which play a critical role in maintaining a healthy immune system. A healthy gut can help to improve the immune system by producing hormones that regulate the immune system and by maintaining a balanced microbiome. A strong immune system can help to protect against infections, diseases, and other health problems.

Conclusion:

In conclusion, a healthy gut-heart-brain connection has numerous benefits for overall health. By prioritizing gut health, we can improve the health of our heart and brain, reduce inflammation, improve digestion and nutrient absorption, and strengthen the immune system. By incorporating a healthy diet, regular exercise, stress management, and probiotics and upplements into our daily routine, we can support the health of the gut and achieve optimal health. By focusing on gut health, we can improve our overall wellbeing and reduce the risk of various health problems.

Chapter 9: Maintaining a Healthy Gut-Heart-Brain Connection

Introduction:

In this chapter, we will discuss practical steps that can be taken to maintain a healthy gut-heart-brain connection. By incorporating these steps into our daily routine, we can improve gut health, reduce the risk of chronic diseases, and enhance overall health and wellbeing.

Healthy Diet:

A healthy diet is essential for maintaining a healthy gut-heart-brain connection. A diet rich in fiber, fruits, vegetables, and whole grains can help to support the health of the gut microbiome and reduce the risk of chronic diseases. Avoiding processed foods, added sugars, and unhealthy fats can also help to improve gut health.

Regular Exercise:

Regular exercise is important for maintaining a healthy gut-heart-brain connection. Exercise can help to reduce stress, improve digestion, and regulate hormones that regulate inflammation and the immune system. Aim for at least 30 minutes of moderate-intensity exercise most days of the week.

Stress Management:

Stress can have a negative impact on gut health and increase the risk of chronic diseases. Stress management techniques, such as meditation, yoga, and deep breathing, can help to reduce stress and improve gut health.

Probiotics and Supplements:

Probiotics and supplements can help to support the health of the gut microbiome and improve gut health. Probiotics can help to maintain a balanced microbiome, while supplements, such as prebiotics, can help to feed the beneficial bacteria in the gut. Consult with a healthcare provider to determine the best probiotics and supplements for your needs.

Conclusion:

In conclusion, maintaining a healthy gut-heart-brain connection requires a combination of a healthy diet, regular exercise, stress management, and probiotics and supplements. By incorporating these steps into our daily routine, we can improve gut health, reduce the risk of chronic diseases, and enhance overall health and wellbeing. By focusing on gut health, we can improve our overall wellbeing and reduce the risk of various health problems. By taking care of our gut, we can support the health of our heart and brain and achieve optimal health and wellbeing.

Chapter 10: Addressing Gut Health Concerns

Introduction:

In this chapter, we will discuss common gut health concerns and how to address them. A healthy gut is essential for maintaining a healthy gut-heart-brain connection, and addressing gut health concerns can help to improve overall health and wellbeing.

Digestive Issues:

Digestive issues, such as bloating, constipation, and diarrhea, can be a sign of poor gut health. These issues can be addressed by incorporating a healthy diet, regular exercise, and stress management into your daily routine. Probiotics and supplements can also help to improve digestive health.

Leaky Gut Syndrome:

Leaky gut syndrome is a condition in which the gut becomes permeable, allowing harmful substances to enter the bloodstream. This can result in inflammation and a range of health problems. Leaky gut syndrome can be addressed by incorporating a healthy diet, reducing stress, and taking probiotics and supplements.

Small Intestinal Bacterial Overgrowth (SIBO):

SIBO is a condition in which bacteria overgrow in the small intestine, leading to digestive problems and nutrient deficiencies. SIBO can be addressed by incorporating a healthy diet, reducing stress, and taking probiotics and supplements. Antibiotics may also be prescribed to help eliminate the overgrowth of bacteria.

Food Intolerances:

Food intolerances can result in digestive problems and inflammation. Common food intolerances include lactose and gluten intolerance. Food intolerances can be addressed by eliminating the offending food from your diet and incorporating a healthy diet, regular exercise, and stress management into your daily routine.

Conclusion:

In conclusion, addressing gut health concerns is essential for maintaining a healthy gut-heart-brain connection. By incorporating a healthy diet, regular exercise, stress management, and probiotics and supplements into your daily routine, you can improve gut health and reduce the risk of various health problems. If you experience digestive problems or other gut health concerns, it is important to seek the advice of a healthcare provider to determine the best course of action. By taking care of our gut, we can support the health of our heart and brain and achieve optimal health and wellbeing.

Chapter 11: The Importance of a Healthy Lifestyle for Gut Health

Introduction:

In this chapter, we will discuss the importance of a healthy lifestyle for maintaining a healthy gut-heart-brain connection. A healthy lifestyle can help to improve gut health and reduce the risk of various health problems.

Diet:

A healthy diet is essential for maintaining a healthy gut. Incorporating a variety of fruits, vegetables, whole grains, and lean proteins into your diet can help to improve gut health. Additionally, reducing processed foods, sugar, and unhealthy fats can help to reduce inflammation and support gut health.

Exercise:

Regular exercise is important for maintaining a healthy gut-heart-brain connection. Exercise can help to improve gut function, reduce inflammation, and support overall health and wellbeing. Aim to exercise for at least 30 minutes a day, five days a week.

Stress Management:

Stress can have a negative impact on gut health, leading to digestive problems and inflammation. Incorporating stress management techniques, such as meditation, yoga, and deep breathing, can help to reduce stress and improve gut health.

Sleep:

Adequate sleep is important for maintaining a healthy gut-heart-brain connection. Lack of sleep can lead to inflammation and digestive problems. Aim to get at least 7-8 hours of sleep per night to support gut health.

Conclusion:

In conclusion, a healthy lifestyle is essential for maintaining a healthy gut-heart-brain connection. By incorporating a healthy diet, regular exercise, stress management, and adequate sleep into your daily routine, you can improve gut health and reduce the risk of various health problems. By taking care of our gut, we can support the health of our heart and brain and achieve optimal health and wellbeing.

Chapter 12: The Future of Gut Health Research and Treatments

Introduction:

In this chapter, we will discuss the future of gut health research and treatments. With the growing understanding of the gut-heart-brain connection, there is a growing interest in developing new treatments and strategies to support gut health.

Probiotics and Prebiotics:

Probiotics and prebiotics are two of the most promising areas of gut health research. Probiotics are beneficial bacteria that can help to improve gut health and reduce the risk of various health problems. Prebiotics are foods that feed the beneficial bacteria in the gut, helping to support their growth and function.

Fecal Microbiota Transplantation (FMT):

Fecal microbiota transplantation (FMT) is a new and promising treatment for digestive problems and other health problems related to the gut-heart-brain connection. FMT involves transplanting healthy gut bacteria from a donor into the gut of a recipient. This treatment has shown promising results in the treatment of various health problems, including inflammatory bowel disease, irritable bowel syndrome, and more.

Personalized Gut Health Treatments:

With the growing understanding of the gut-heart-brain connection, there is a growing interest in developing personalized gut health treatments. These treatments are tailored to the specific needs of each individual, based on their gut microbiome, health history, and other factors. Personalized gut health treatments have the potential to be more effective and efficient than traditional treatments.

Conclusion:

In conclusion, the future of gut health research and treatments is bright. With the growing understanding of the gut-heart-brain connection, there is a growing interest in developing new treatments and strategies to support gut health. Probiotics and prebiotics, fecal microbiota transplantation, and personalized gut health treatments are just a few of the exciting developments in this field. As research continues, we can expect to see even more innovative and effective treatments for gut health and the gut-heart-brain connection in the future.

Chapter 13: The Benefits of an Elimination Diet for Gut Health

Introduction:

In this chapter, we will discuss the benefits of an elimination diet for gut health. An elimination diet is a dietary approach that involves removing certain foods from your diet to identify any food sensitivities or allergies. This approach can be an effective way to improve gut health and support the gut-heart-brain connection.

Identifying Food Sensitivities and Allergies:

An elimination diet can help you identify any food sensitivities or allergies that may be contributing to digestive problems and other health problems related to the gut-heart-brain connection. By removing certain foods from your diet and then gradually reintroducing them, you can identify which foods may be causing problems for you and avoid them in the future.

Improving Gut Health:

An elimination diet can also help to improve gut health by reducing inflammation and promoting the growth of beneficial bacteria in the gut. By avoiding certain foods that may be causing digestive problems or other health problems, you can reduce inflammation in the gut and support the growth of beneficial bacteria. This can help to improve gut health and support the gut-heart-brain connection.

Reducing Symptoms of Digestive Problems:

An elimination diet can also be an effective way to reduce symptoms of digestive problems, such as bloating, gas, constipation, and diarrhea. By avoiding certain foods that may be causing these symptoms, you can reduce or eliminate them and improve your overall gut health.

Improving Overall Health:

In addition to improving gut health, an elimination diet can also have a positive impact on your overall health. By reducing inflammation and promoting the growth of beneficial bacteria in the gut, you can improve your immune system and reduce the risk of various health problems, including heart disease, diabetes, and more.

Conclusion:

In conclusion, an elimination diet can be an effective way to improve gut health and support the gut-heart-brain connection. By identifying food sensitivities and allergies, reducing inflammation, and promoting the growth of beneficial bacteria in the gut, an elimination diet can have a positive impact on your overall health and well-being. If you are experiencing digestive problems or other health problems related to the gut-heart-brain connection, consider trying an elimination diet to see if it can help.

Chapter 14: The Benefits of a Carnivore Diet for Gut Health

Introduction:

In this chapter, we will discuss the benefits of a carnivore diet for gut health and the gut-heart-brain connection. The carnivore diet is a dietary approach that involves consuming only animal products, such as meat, fish, and dairy, and avoiding all plant-based foods, including carbohydrates. This approach has become increasingly popular in recent years as a way to improve gut health and support the gut-heart-brain connection.

Reducing Inflammation:

One of the key benefits of a carnivore diet is its ability to reduce inflammation in the body. Inflammation is a natural response to injury or infection, but chronic inflammation can contribute to a range of health problems, including heart disease, diabetes, and more. By avoiding plant-based foods that are high in carbohydrates and can cause inflammation, a carnivore diet can help to reduce inflammation in the body and support the gut-heart-brain connection.

Improving Gut Health:

Another benefit of a carnivore diet is its ability to improve gut health. Animal products are rich in nutrients that are essential for gut health, including protein, healthy fats, and vitamins and minerals. By consuming these nutrients in their purest form, a carnivore diet can help to support the growth of beneficial bacteria in the gut and improve gut health.

Promoting Weight Loss:

In addition to improving gut health, a carnivore diet can also promote weight loss. By eliminating carbohydrates and focusing on high-protein, high-fat foods, a carnivore diet can help you feel fuller for longer and reduce your overall calorie intake. This can lead to weight loss and improved health.

Improving Heart Health:

A carnivore diet can also have a positive impact on heart health. By reducing inflammation and promoting weight loss, a carnivore diet can help to reduce the risk of heart disease and other cardiovascular problems. Additionally, the high-protein, high-fat foods consumed on a carnivore diet can help to improve cholesterol levels and support heart health.

Conclusion:

In conclusion, a carnivore diet can be a beneficial approach for improving gut health and supporting the gut-heart-brain connection. By reducing inflammation, promoting weight loss, and improving heart health, a carnivore diet can have a positive impact on your overall health and well-being. However, it is important to note that a carnivore diet may not be suitable for everyone, and it is important to consult with a healthcare professional before starting any new dietary approach.

Chapter 15: The Dangers of Overconsumption of Fiber

Introduction:

In this chapter, we will discuss the dangers of overconsumption of fiber for gut health and the gut-heart-brain connection. While fiber is widely recognized as an important component of a healthy diet, consuming too much fiber can have negative effects on gut health and the gut-heart-brain connection.

Damage to Intestinal Villi:

One of the main dangers of overconsumption of fiber is the damage it can cause to the intestinal villi. These tiny finger-like projections in the intestines are responsible for absorbing nutrients from food. When too much fiber is consumed, it can cause the villi to become damaged and less effective at absorbing nutrients. This can lead to malabsorption and malnutrition, as the body is not able to absorb the nutrients it needs to function properly.

Impact on Gut Microbiome:

Another danger of overconsumption of fiber is its impact on the gut microbiome. The gut microbiome is a complex community of bacteria, yeast, and other microorganisms that play a crucial role in gut health and the gut-heart-brain connection. When too much fiber is consumed, it can disrupt the delicate balance of the gut microbiome, leading to an overgrowth of harmful bacteria and a reduction in beneficial bacteria. This can contribute to a range of health problems, including digestive issues, inflammation, and more.

Increased Risk of Gut Inflammation:

Overconsumption of fiber can also increase the risk of gut inflammation. Inflammation is a natural response to injury or infection, but chronic inflammation can contribute to a range of health problems, including heart disease, diabetes, and more. By consuming too much fiber, you can increase the risk of gut inflammation, which can have negative effects on gut health and the gut-heart-brain connection.

Conclusion:

In conclusion, while fiber is an important component of a healthy diet, overconsumption of fiber can have negative effects on gut health and the gut-heart-brain connection. By causing damage to the intestinal villi, impacting the gut microbiome, and increasing the risk of gut inflammation, overconsumption of fiber can lead to malabsorption and malnutrition. It is important to consume fiber in moderation and to work with a healthcare professional to determine the right amount of fiber for your individual needs.

Chapter 16: The Simple Importance of Sleep

Introduction:

In this chapter, we will discuss the importance of sleep for gut health and the gut-heart-brain connection. Sleep is a crucial aspect of overall health and wellness, and it plays a key role in maintaining the delicate balance of the gut-heart-brain connection.

Impact on Gut Microbiome:

Sleep has a significant impact on the gut microbiome, which is a complex community of bacteria, yeast, and other microorganisms that play a crucial role in gut health and the gut-heart-brain connection. Sleep deprivation can disrupt the delicate balance of the gut microbiome, leading to an overgrowth of harmful bacteria and a reduction in beneficial bacteria. This can contribute to a range of health problems, including digestive issues, inflammation, and more.

Influence on Digestion:

Sleep also has a significant influence on digestion. During sleep, the body produces hormones that regulate digestion, including the release of digestive enzymes and the regulation of gut motility. Sleep deprivation can disrupt this delicate hormonal balance, leading to digestive issues such as bloating, constipation, and more.

Impact on Mental Health:

Sleep also plays a crucial role in mental health, which is closely tied to the gut-heart-brain connection. Sleep deprivation can contribute to a range of mental health problems, including anxiety, depression, and more. By getting enough sleep, you can help maintain a healthy gut-heart-brain connection and protect against these mental health problems.

Conclusion:

In conclusion, sleep is an important aspect of overall health and wellness, and it plays a key role in maintaining the delicate balance of the gut-heart-brain connection. By impacting the gut microbiome, influencing digestion, and impacting mental health, sleep is a crucial component of gut health. It is important to prioritize sleep and aim for 7-9 hours of quality sleep each night to maintain a healthy gut-heart-brain connection.

Chapter 17: Stress Management for Gut Health and the Gut-Heart-Brain Connection

Introduction:

In this chapter, we will discuss the importance of stress management for gut health and the gut-heart-brain connection. Stress is a natural part of life, but when it becomes chronic, it can have a significant impact on our health, including our gut health and the gut-heart-brain connection.

Impact on Gut Microbiome:

Stress can have a significant impact on the gut microbiome, which is a complex community of bacteria, yeast, and other microorganisms that play a crucial role in gut health and the gut-heart-brain connection. Chronic stress can disrupt the delicate balance of the gut microbiome, leading to an overgrowth of harmful bacteria and a reduction in beneficial bacteria. This can contribute to a range of health problems, including digestive issues, inflammation, and more.

Influence on Digestion:

Stress also has a significant influence on digestion. When we experience stress, our bodies release hormones such as cortisol, which can disrupt digestive function and lead to issues such as bloating, constipation, and more. By managing stress, we can help maintain a healthy gut-heart-brain connection and protect against these digestive issues.

Impact on Mental Health:

Stress also plays a crucial role in mental health, which is closely tied to the gut-heart-brain connection. Chronic stress can contribute to a range of mental health problems, including anxiety, depression, and more. By managing stress, you can help maintain a healthy gut-heart-brain connection and protect against these mental health problems.

Stress Management Techniques:

There are many effective stress management techniques that can help you maintain a healthy gut-heart-brain connection. These techniques include exercise, mindfulness, deep breathing, journaling, and more. It is important to find what works best for you and make stress management a regular part of your routine.

Conclusion:

In conclusion, stress management is an important aspect of overall health and wellness, and it plays a key role in maintaining the delicate balance of the gut-heart-brain connection. By impacting the gut microbiome, influencing digestion, and impacting mental health, stress is a crucial component of gut health. It is important to prioritize stress management and make it a regular part of your routine to maintain a healthy gut-heart-brain connection.

Chapter 18: The Future of Gut Health and the Gut-Heart-Brain Connection

As research in the field of gut health continues to advance, the importance of the gut-heart-brain connection is becoming increasingly clear. In the future, we can expect to see more personalized approaches to gut health, based on individual factors such as genetics, diet, and lifestyle.

One promising area of research is the use of probiotics and prebiotics to improve gut health. Probiotics are live bacteria and yeasts that are beneficial to the gut, while prebiotics are non-digestible fibers that feed the good bacteria in the gut. Studies have shown that taking probiotics and prebiotics can improve gut health and reduce inflammation, which in turn can have positive effects on heart and brain health.

Another area of research is the use of fecal microbiota transplants (FMTs) to treat gut-related disorders. FMTs involve transplanting healthy gut bacteria from one person to another, and have been shown to be effective in treating conditions such as irritable bowel syndrome and Clostridium difficile infections.

In addition to these treatments, there will likely be a greater emphasis on lifestyle changes to improve gut health in the future. This may include changes to diet, such as reducing the intake of processed foods and increasing the consumption of fiber-rich foods, as well as changes to physical activity and stress management practices.

Ultimately, the future of gut health and the gut-heart-brain connection is bright, and we can expect to see continued advancements in our understanding of how the gut affects our overall health and well-being. By taking care of our gut, we can improve our heart and brain health and live a happier, healthier life.

Epilogue: The Power of Gut Health

As you've learned throughout this book, the gut-heart-brain connection is a complex and interrelated system that is crucial for our overall health and well-being. By taking care of our gut, we can improve our heart and brain health, reduce inflammation, and lead a happier, healthier life.

While there is still much to learn about the gut-heart-brain connection, the evidence is clear that gut health is essential for our overall health. Whether you're looking to improve your digestion, boost your immune system, or simply feel better, taking care of your gut is a great place to start.

There are many ways to improve gut health, from changing your diet and lifestyle to taking probiotics and prebiotics. Whatever approach you choose, the most important thing is to listen to your body and make changes that work for you.

As we move into the future, we can expect to see continued advancements in our understanding of the gut-heart-brain connection and the role of gut health in our overall health. Whether you're a healthcare professional or simply someone who wants to live a healthier life, it's never been a better time to learn about the power of gut health.

So take the first step today, and start taking care of your gut. Your heart and brain will thank you!

www.ingramcontent.com/pod-product-compliance
Lightning Source LLC
Chambersburg PA
CBHW060949130726

48001CB00003B/1138